Essential Oils for Depression

Essential Oil Recipes for
Depression
for Diffusers, Roller Bottles,
Inhalers & more.

Rica V. Gadi

Printed in the United States of America

First Printing, 2019

ISBN: 9781793029393

http://eorecipes.net

DISCLAIMER: This document is a compilation of recipes used successfully by EO enthusiasts who use only high-quality, therapeutic-grade essential oils as determined by many factors including growth, growth location, harvesting process, distillation method used, etc. Please be advised that not all essential oils are created equally, and not all essential oils are suitable for topical use or ingestion. Please do your research before choosing the brand(s) of essential oils you decide to use as well as supplies you use. Always follow label directions on the essential oil bottles.

All the recipes in this book have been inspired by essential oil believers. However, we are not medical practitioners and cannot diagnose, treat or prescribe treatment for any health condition or disease. Just a precaution, before using any alternative medicines, natural supplements, or vitamins, you should always discuss the products you are using or intend to use with your doctor, especially if you are pregnant, trying to get pregnant or nursing.

All information contained within this book is for reference purposes only, and is not intended to substitute advice given by a pharmacist, physician or other licensed health-care professional. As such, the author is not responsible for any loss, claim or damage arising from use of the essential oil recipes contained herein.

This book is dedicated to all the strong people who are taking responsibility of your own well being and doing something to be better.

All my heartfelt gratitude to the following people: my mom Ruby Jane, you have made me everything I am today; my dad Nestor-- my eternal, my angel, and the source of my perseverance; Mommyling, my spiritual guide ; Ria & Joe, the true witnesses of my transformation and my foundation pillars; Ellie Jane, the sparkle of our eyes;

Juan, thanks for always encouraging me to push harder - you are my ONE; Rocco & Radha, my reason for everything.

The Love of my family and friends is the fountain of inspiration that never runs dry. Thank you for constantly inspiring me, motivating me, and loving me unconditionally.

This book will never be complete without the help of my trusted and talented friends the #NOWsuperstars and my #oilbularya friends

Blending Essential Oils to use for a very specific reason has become very popular in the recent years. There are several reasons why this is so. Blending EOs is basically about inhaling - as it has been proven that aromas have the ability to trigger feelings, emotions and personal memories.

With this in mind, it is obvious that everyone is unique when it comes to what triggers your senses. It all boils down to personal preference for the aroma to trigger what you want to unleash. Everyone is different and we all connect to the aroma differently, so what might work for one might not work for another person.

Of course, we also want the blend we personalize to be therapeutic. This is the best reason why to blend essential oils. We want the blend we create to help us with a very specific emotion or physical condition. As much as smelling good is important in a blend, it is more important that we blend oils that is not only pleasing to the smell but also produces the therapeutic effect we are after.

Then you have to think about contraindications. Making sure the blend you create is safe to use.

I suggest that before blending find out if the oils you are using is safe for a condition you may have example, if you are pregnant, or have specific allergies. Consult your physician prior to moving forward.

The recipes I have in this book is a compilation of what has proven to work and favored by hundreds of EO enthusiasts. It takes out the guesswork to get you started.

Again, we urge you to read the recipes and make sure that this is safe for you to try.

The book is very specific to a physical and emotional condition. There are several recipes here because you might want to rotate and you may like one and not the other. There is also a variety of application. Some of us prefer to diffuse, some to make roller bottles, and others to create sprays.

I hope you enjoy this compilation, feel free to use the notes section and jot down your fave blends. There is a wonderful world of EO blending - this is just the beginning.

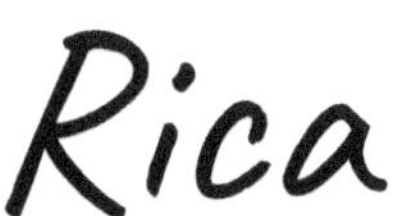

Depression is super hard to pinpoint and it is such a complex condition because there is not one definite cause that we can identify or associate with it. There can be multiple reasons why depression happens. It could be coming from a life events or a sudden change of life pattern or something more serious like fatal illnesses. This disease come without warning, it just dawns on you and suddenly you are overwhelmed with extreme loneliness or sadness without explanation.

Depression is a mental health issue that is common globally. Although it is all in the mind, it has the ability to affect your physical well-being as well. Symptoms that go along with depression may include one of the following:

- Extreme Sadness
- Feeling of Emptiness
- Memory Loss
- Obsession with death
- Increased Heart Rate or Heart Attack Risk
- Weight Changes
- Blood Vessels are Constricted
- Heightened Sensitivity to Pain
- Fatigue
- Decreased Libido
- Immune System is Weak

Depression becomes a concern because sometimes when people are depressed they resort to using drugs or excessive alcohol consumption, this greatly increases the chances of reckless behaviors or abusive habits. Also, during depressive moments is when most people have thoughts of suicide or inflicting pain to themselves.

Essential oils have been known to be effective in helping treat depression, as a gamut of evidences have been presented over the years to support that. It has been known to help uplift your spirits and elevate your mood safely and naturally. It can also aid in relieving feelings of stress and anxiety, which usually come with depression.

Essential oils have the capacity to bring forth feelings of Joy, Increased Energy, Calming and Relaxation. It also has some physical abilities like improving your blood circulation and promote hormonal balance.

Depression affect millions of people worldwide and it is not something we freely share with the people around us. It is important that we can take action and find a way out but it i also advisable that when you suspect that you are in the state of depression, to seek expert and medical opinion so they may be able to guide you in this journey and can advice you about the administration of Essential Oils into your daily routine.

With depression it is always wise to first ge[t] appropriate medical advice as soon as early signs manifest itself. You have nothing to lose and everything to gain, as only the experts know how to detect these. Everybody gets sad at some point but when you feel these symptoms, it doesn't hurt to see your physician

- Feeling of hopelessness almost daily that last[s] a week or more
- Extreme sadness for an entire day, for a series of consecutive days
- Loss of interest in activities you normally enjoy like : hanging out with friends, playing sports hobbies
- Harboring feelings of guilt, worthlessness and helplessness
- Thoughts of harming yourself or committing suicide, attempt to do either
- Your sleep patterns changes drastically
- Sudden change of weight
- Feelings of extreme fatigue for an entire day
- No Energy for Daily routinely activities
- Uncontrollable crying without reason
- Difficulty in Focusing, Making decisions or memory loss
- Persistent pains in your body and migraines/headaches
- Feelings of restlessness, irritability and constant annoyance

Remember, you are not alone and someone cars, you just have to reach out and ask for it. It is OK and it happens.

Table of Contents

Fight Depression with Essential Oils

Depression can hit you at any point of your life and the best alternative is the use of Essential oils. For some people, depression develops later on in life. For other people, they are chronically incapacitated from depression since they were children. Regardless of when depression began in your life, it is important to do something to help boost your self-esteem and rid your life from depression. Depression can cause anxiety and it can ultimately cause you to become unhealthy and physically harm your body.

Depression comes in all different types, forms, and it can be rare outbreaks or it can be a looming cloud over a severely depressed person. Essential oils for depression can help you overcome depression in your life, and it can give you a boost in attitude and a complete overhaul in how you view your life. The aromatherapy is a natural way to help you balance mood swings and deal with debilitating depression. Some people use drugs and other chemicals to deal with depression. These drugs have unknown side effects, and they can occasionally become a negative impact on the mind. Aromatherapy is completely natural and it is a safe way to battle depression which has been used for thousands of years.

Not only is depression bad for your mental health, but it can eventually affect your physical health as well. Depression is also cause stress and stress is a well-known killer for people who keep emotions inside. Depression can cause social anxiety and health issues. It can be the cause of a loss of appetite, mood swings, and you can lose your job over severe depression. These are reasons why depression should be contained and dealt with quickly before it becomes out of hand.

Other natural ways to assist essential oils for depression in eliminating the dilemma is daily exercise, efficient nightly stress, and a boost in self-confidence. Essential oils in aromatherapy can help, but coupled with the above activities you can find your depression slowly fading. Essential oils can help you fight off depression effectively without all the drugs and chemicals. Aromatherapy penetrates the senses and helps you fight off the negative effects of depression with stimulating fragrances and scents.

The following essential oils for depression are powerful solutions to help fight off depression. Jasmine, Lavender, and Neroli are three essential oils that will successfully boost your mood and help you balance your emotions. The essential oils can be used separately for their individual benefits to help you fight depression. Use them together as a potent solutions to help rid yourself from depression quickly and efficiently.

Jasmine

Jasmine is a sensual essential oil for depression that helps you assert yourself. It can relax you beyond the stressful day and it can lift your emotions. It can also boost your confidence and your self-esteem to help overcome the controversy from the day.

Lavender French

Lavender French is a soothing essential oil for depression that can help you mentally relax. It is an herb from France that has become popular for its therapeutic uses. It can help balance your mood and release the tension from your mind and your muscles.

Neroli

Neroli is a popular relaxing and rejuvenating essential oil for depression. Its fragrance is incredibly relaxing and it can help you dispel anger and irritability. Use this essential oil to help you have a good night's sleep and help you feel refreshed.

All-natural therapies that can calm the nerves and mind are capable of relieving anxiety and stress. When it comes to essential oils for depression, there is no fixed combination and what works for one person won't necessarily work for another. Since everyone is biochemically exclusive, it is advisable to experiment with several essential oils, pay close attention to your body, and find the right blend that works optimally for you and your body.

It is also worth mentioning that the following oils are worth checking out for Migraines **Bergamot, Lavender, Ylang Ylang, Grapefruit, Chamomile, Sandalwood, Basil, Orange, Clary Sage, Geranium, Turmeric, Rose and Cedarwood**

The Blending Process

These EOs are categorized by aromas, and EOs from the same group usually blend fantastically together.

- Floral – Lavender, Geranium, Jasmine
- Woodsy – Pine, Cedarwood
- Earthy – Vetiver, Patchouli
- Herbaceous – Marjoram, Rosemary, Basil
- Minty – Peppermint, Spearmint, Wintergreen
- Medicinal – Eucalyptus, Frankincense, Melaleuca
- Spicy – Pepper, Clove, Cinnamon
- Oriental – Ginger, Patchouli
- Citrus – Wild Orange, Lemon, Lime

Select oils that will give you with the health benefits you are looking to remedy. For increased energy choose: Grapefruit, Lemon, Orange, or Citrus. For Calming and Relaxation choose: Lavender, Cedarwood, or Chamomile. You are encouraged to experiment and play with your oils to see which blends work for you.

TIPS:

- Combine Floral EOs with Woodsy, Spicy and Citrus aromas
- Minty EOs with Woodsy, Earthy, Herbaceous and Citrus aromas
- Earthy EOs with Woodsy and Minty aromas
- Citrus EOs with Floral, Woodsy, Minty, Spicy and Oriental aromas

Diffuse

Diffusing Essential Oils is the safest method to enjoy Essential Oils without the risk of an allergic reaction.

Diffusing Essential Oils
Some Tidbits You Need To Know

Our sense of smell is one of our most powerful senses, and as you have noticed in your own experience that some scents affect your more positively in your minds than others. The body contains over 1,000 receptors for smell—way more receptors than for any of our other senses.

Diffusion Essential Oils means the process vaporizes oils into air by releasing tiny amounts into the air. Inhalation is totally safe and is super low risk. Chances of any EO rising to dangerous levels while diffusion is slim to none.

Diffusing Essential Oils around newborns, babies, young children, pregnant or nursing women, and pets should be done with caution. Read up on safety.

It is advisable that Diffusing Essential Oils for only about 15-30 minutes at a time to be most effective. NEVER leave your diffuser on overnight. Make sure your diffuser is filled with the right amount of water and you understand the operating directions.

While diffusing essential oils, be sure that your space has great ventilation. Crack a window open if the scent become to strong.

Never add Carrier Oils to your diffuser. This may cause your diffuser to malfunction. Clean your diffuser at least 3 times a week with warm water and natural soap to ensure the diffuser is well maintained and bacteria and mold does not accumulate.

Diffusing Essential Oils Basic Guidelines

Just a few things you need to know and prepare before getting started Diffusing Essential Oils.

Things you need:
Ultrasonic Oil Diffuser
Essential Oils
Water

Just follow the number of drops in the recipe, drop on to an oil diffuser and fill the rest with water.

All diffusers are different and will have its own water minimum and maximum level. Read the diffuser instruction before use.

Ideally, it is best to diffuse for 15-30 minutes and turn off the diffuser. The effect should be good for at least 2-3 hours. Turn your diffuser back on after 3 hours to reinforce oil diffusing effects.

It is not advisable to use EO in humidifiers.These are not made to release EOS

Diffuser Recipes

Here's a thought for you:

You may be wondering how aroma can simply eliminate symptoms. There's a simple answer to this : Aroma is simply a by-product of diffusing. It's the added benefit but in reality the real benefit comes from the air we breathe and how the body easily absorbs the essential oils released in the air. It works 2 ways, not only does it improve the air quality you breath by disinfecting and eliminating pollutants it also allows your glands to absorb the healing elements of the EOs released in the air molecules,

So for here are a few recipes that can help you manage symptoms and actual issues regarding the matter :

4 Drops Spearmint
3 Drops Tangerine

----

4 Drops Grapefruit
3 Drops Fennel

----

2 Drops Lavender
2 Drops Wild Orange
2 Drops Wintergreen
2 Drops White Fir

----

4 Drops Bergamot
4 Drops White Angelica

----

2 Drops Frankincense
2 Drops Orange
2 Drops Lavender

----

2 Drops Frankincense
2 Drops Bergamot
2 Drops Orange

----

4 Drops Orange
2 Drops Lavender
1 Drop Ylang Ylang

----

3 Drops Neroli
3 Drops Sweet Orange
1 Drop Frankincense
1 Drop Lemon
1 Drop Ylang Ylang

----

2 Drops Wild Orange
2 Drops Bergamot
2 Drops Cypress
2 Drops Frankincense

----

3 Drops Lavender
3 Drops Bergamot

----

3 Drops Peppermint
3 Drops Lemon
2 Drops Orange

----

4 Drops Lavender
2 Drops Lemon
2 Drops Ylang Ylang

----

4 Drops Lavender
3 Drops Chamomile

----

2 Drops Frankincense
2 Drops Bergamot
2 Drops Orange

----

3 Drops Bergamot
2 Drops Lavender
2 Drops Clary Sage
1 Drop Ylang Ylang

----

4 Drops Lavender
2 Drops Vetiver

----

4 Drops Orange
2 Drops Lavender
1 Drop Ylang Ylang

----

3 Drops Rosemary
3 Drops Peppermint
3 Drops Lemon

----

2 Drops Grapefruit
3 Drops Peppermint
3 Drops Rosemary

----

3 Drops Wild Orange
3 Drops Frankincense
2 Drops Cinnamon

----

3 Drops Grapefruit
3 Drops Joy

----

3 Drops Stress Away
3 Drops Peppermint

----

4 Drops Peppermint
5 Drops Sweet Orange

----

35 Drops Rosemary
3 Drops Grapefruit
3 Drops Lime

----

3 Drops Sweet Orange
3 Drops Grapefruit
2 Drops Lemon
1 Drop Bergamot

----

3 Drops Peppermint
3 Drops Lemon
2 Drops Orange

----

2 Drops Wild Orange
2 Drops Frankincense
2 Drops Cinnamon

----

2 Drops Eucalyptus
2 Drops Geranium
1 Drop Lemon
1 Drop Thyme

Roll

Essential Oil Roller Bottles is the easiest method to enjoy Essential Oils Anywhere and Whenever.

Blending Essential Oils in a Roller Bottle
Some Tidbits You Need To Know

Essential Oils are usually super concentrated and too hard to measure how much to actually put straight from the bottle.

Roller bottles are a way that you are able to create blends ready to use with the right dilution. It allows your EO to last longer.

It also makes it easier to apply exactly where you want to target without getting it all over the place.

It is handy and easy to carry in your purse, ready to use at any time you want to.

I like to apply EOs at the bottom of the feet for many reasons. Our feet have bigger pores than any other skin in our bodies. this means that they are able to suck in the therapeutic compounds in our blend into the bloodstream faster that any other parts of the body. Imagine comparing a normal straw to an oversized straw and how much more you can suck in with the latter. This is how the soles of our feet is compared to the rest of the skin in our bodies.

The skin on our feet is also less sensitive and is designed to withstand some abuse. The risk of having an irritation from EOS is less likely to happen when applied on the feet.

The feet don't have the glands that act as a barrier. Sebaceous glands are glands in our skin that produces an oily substance called Sebum, for the purpose of lubricating and waterproofing the skin. Since this is oil and if you put oil on top of oil, it can act as a barrier or it may slow down penetration.

The feet and palms of our hands are the only skin that don't have these, so it is ideal to apply Essential Oils to the feet for maximum penetration.

Now, it would be hard to apply oils directly and very mess, right? Roller bottles make it super easy and convenient to roll the EOs at the bottom of our feet.

Carrier Oils Info

Carrier oils are vegetable-based oils with their own healing properties that dilute essential oils used to help carry the EOs into the skin.

Essential oils are highly concentrated and could evaporate very quickly. The carrier oil is mixed with the essential oil so it could penetrate the skin before it actually evaporates. Although EOs are oils, it is actually not that oily. When mixed with a carrier oil, it allows you to have more of the essential oil into your skin without wasting EOS to evaporate, making the healing properties of the EO strong and more effective.

There are also Essential oils that are too strong to apply directly to the skin and may cause damage, so it is important to dilute them with a carrier oil.

Never add Carrier Oils to your diffuser. This may cause your diffuser to malfunction. Clean your diffuser at least 3 times a week with warm water and natural soap to ensure the diffuser is well maintained and bacteria and mold does not accumulate.

Carrier Oils

There are a lot of different carrier oils that you can use with EOs to dilute them in a roller bottle.

To name a few :

Almond Oil - moisturizing and stays liquid at room temperature. Do not use if you are allergic to nuts.

Apricot Kernel Oil - moisturizing and suitable for sensitive skin or kids. It is super gentle on the skin.

Avocado Oil - moisturizing and suitable for sensitive and damaged skin. Perfect for skin problems.Can be mixed with other carrier oils

Castor Oil - with antibacterial, antiviral and antifungal properties, use topically to eliminate pain and relieve skin irritation.

Coconut Oil - its antibacterial, antiviral and antifungal properties it is the best and most versatile for skin care. The skin absorbs this very quickly. It solidifies in room temp and may still have a slight coconut oil aroma in it - but you can get a fractionated coconut oil to eliminate the 2 challenges above.

Grapeseed Oil - not just for cooking but also great for topical application on the skin.

Jojoba Oil - one of my faves for skin care blends. This oil is the closest to our natural oil our skin produces to it is absorbed easily without being oily. Also amazing for massage oil blends.

Olive Oil - this is the oil for herb type oils. mostly used for cooking but can also be applied to the skin but would need to be blended with a carrier oil that is mild and absorb well with the skin.

Rosehip Seed Oil - super good for deep moisturizing or skin irritations. This oil has a high content of antioxidants and helps remedy dry, scarred and wounded skin.

Recommended Roller Bottle Dilution Guide

RECOMMENDED ROLL-ON BOTTLE DILUTION AMOUNTS

5 ml (1/6 oz.) Roll-on Bottle = ~100 drops (1tsp.)
10 ml (1/3 oz.) Roll-on Bottle = ~200 drops (2 tsp.)
30 ml. (1 oz.) Roll-on Bottle = ~600 drops (6 tsp.)

Roll-on Size	5 ml	10 ml	30 ml	Add EO drops to roll-on, then fill with carrier oil.	Dilution Percentage
	1	2	6	1%	
	2	4	12	2%	
	3	6	18	3%	
	5	10	30	5%	
Essential Oil Drops	10	20	60	10%	
	20	40	120	20%	
	25	50	150	25%	
	50	100	300	50%	

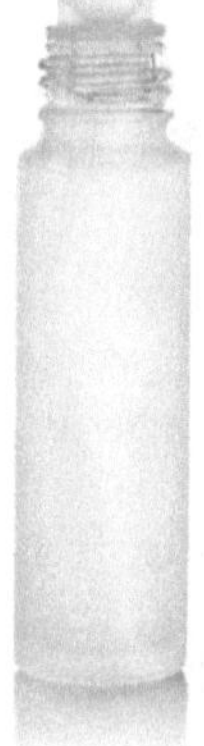
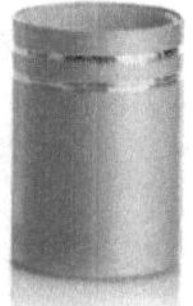

General Guidelines:
Birth to 12 months = .3-.5% dilution
1-5 years = 1.5-3% dilution
6-11 years = 1.5-5% dilution
12-17 years = 1.5-20% dilution
18 years and older = 1.5% dilution-Neat (no dilution)
Elderly or Sensitive Skin = 1-3% dilution
Daily Use = 2-5% dilution
Short Term Use = 10-25% dilution
Local Skin or Systemic Issues = 50% dilution-Neat

These are general guidelines suggestions--not absolute rules--based on traditional aromatheraphy practice.
(Kurt Schnaubelt PhD, Valerie Worwood, Robert Tisserand)

Dilution Basics:

How much you dilute your EO depends on different factors such as weight, sensitivity, health conditions, EOs that are blended in or how long that blend has been used for. There is never an absolute dilution rule, it is you who knows about your level and tolerance. I feel that it is best to start with a higher dilution percentage and increase EO drops over time.

To make sure your EO is safe, make sure that the oils you use are therapeutic grade and do your research on the source and extraction methods used to produce the oils.

Roller Bottle Blending Order

I normally just start with dropping the drops of oils into the **10mL roller bottle**, then adding the carrier oil up until the shoulder of the bottle. Capping the bottle off with the roller and the bottle cap. Instead of shaking the bottle, i like to roll the bottle between my palms first for a minute or 2 for blending, then finishing it off with a few shakes.

NOTE: All recipes in this book is for a 10mL Roller Bottle. If you have a bigger or smaller roller bottle, adjust the number of EO drops based on the size of your bottle.

Roller Bottle Recipes

1 drops Patchouli
1 drops Vetiver
1 drops Lime
5 drops Balance
5 drops Lavender

----

4 drops Joy
3 drops Frankincense
3 drops Orange

----

4 drops Lavender
3 drops Clary sage
2 drops Ylang Ylang
1 drops Marjoram

----

5 drops Valor
4 drops Frankincense
4 drops Lavender
4 drops Cedarwood

----

2 drops White Angelica
2 drops Bergamot
2 drops Valor
2 drops Orange
1 drops Citrus Fresh

----

10 drops Lemon
4 drops Eucalyptus Radiata
3 drops Peppermint
1 drop Cinnamon

----

2 drops Patchouli
2 drops Elevation
2 drops Cedarwood
2 drops Balance
2 drops Basil
2 drops Vetiver

----

6 drops Lime
3 drops Lemon
2 drops Peppermint

----

6 drops Rosemary
4 drops Peppermint
4 drops Grapefruit

----

6 drops White Angelica
6 drops Stress Away

----

8 drops Orange
4 drops Cardamom
3 drops Thieves

----

4 drops Grapefruit
4 drops Wild Orange
3 drops Lemon
2 drops Bergamot

----

2 drops Joy
3 drops Peppermint
4 drops Lemon
4 drops Tangerine

----

4 drops Grapefruit
2 drops Peppermint
2 drops Rosemary
2 drops Thyme

----

5 drops Bergamot
5 drops Frankincense

----

1 drops Patchouli
1 drops Vetiver
1 drops Lime
5 drops Balance
5 drops Lavender

----

7 drops Eucalyptus Radiata
5 drops Rosemary
3 drops Grapefruit

----

3 drops Frankincense
3 drops Bergamot
2 drops Orange
2 drops Grapefruit
2 drops Clary Sage

----

5 drops Eucalyptus
5 drops Spearmint

----

2 drops Orange
2 drops Lemon
2 drops Grapefruit
2 drops Bergamot
4 drops Clary Sage
4 drops Frankincense

----

2 drops Sandalwood
2 drops Ylang Ylang
2 drops Cypress
2 drops Bergamot
2 drops Black Pepper

----

3 drops Black Pepper
3 drops Lime
3 drops Wild Orange
3 drops Frankincense

----

7 drops Eucalyptus
5 drops Rosemary
3 drops Grapefruit

----

4 drops Bergamot
3 drops Wild Orange
2 drops Geranium
2 drops White Fir

----

3 drops Spruce
3 drops Cedarwood
2 drops Juniper Berry
2 drops White Fir

----

4 drops Lavender
3 drops Lemon
2 drops Rosemary
1 drop Cinnamon

Bonus Recipes

Pain Relief Massage Oil Favorite

60mL Jojoba Oil (cold pressed)
8 drops Lavender
8 drops Peppermint
15 drops Frankincense

Pain Relief Massage Oil Secret

14 drops Frankincense
10 drops Sweet Orange
8 drops Turmeric
30mL Sweet Almond Oil

Pain Relief Bath Soak Blend

10 drops Frankincense
5 drops Lavender
5 drops Bergamot
1 cup Full-Cream/ Full-Fat Milk

Pain Relief Bath Salt Blend

1 cup Epsom Salt
¼ cup Dead Sea Salt
¼ cup Baking Soda
8-10 drops Essential Oils
(use any ingredient above or single oils)

Inhale

Essential Oil Inhalers are the most convenient way to enjoy Essential Oils Anywhere and Whenever.

Essential Oil Inhalers give you quick and easy access to the vast therapeutic benefits of essential oils.

Blending Essential Oils in an Inhaler
Some Tidbits You Need To Know

EO Inhalers or aroma sticks are compact tubes, with a cotton wick inside and a protective cover, to lock the aroma within.

Your preferred blend of essential oils is absorbed by the cotton wick, and safely enclosed in a tube that that fits inside of the cover. The cover is easily removed for access to the tube to breathe in the aroma. Usually lasts about 3 months, depending on the oil blend used.

I absolutely love these because they encourage me to take a moment during super stressful moments, and just breathe.

It is in times of stress when our breathing patterns often change and taking deep breaths promote a feeling of calm and inner peace. Breath work combined with visualization plus a relaxing inhaler, can offer relief to symptoms of stress and help your body to come back to the state of homeostasis.

Aroma Sticks can be carried in your tiny purse, even compact enough to fit in your pocket. You can enjoy your favorite EOs anywhere and you can use them with discretion.

I love diffusing, and do all the time but not everyone in my space may enjoy the scents I enjoy or they may not benefit from the therapeutic benefits of the EOs I am diffusing - so the inhaler is one way to not only enjoy my choice of blends but to keep in personal not affecting everyone else around me.

Inhalers not only benefits me but also keep those around me safe in case the oils I want to blend may pose a risk to those around me who may have health issue not advised to be exposed to my choice EOs/

When making Aroma Sticks, You may use your chosen EOs at 100% Concentration.

Inhaler Basic Guidelines

Breathe in slow and deep to absorb the EO molecules directly into your olfactory system.

Inhalers are super easy to use. You just remove the cap and inhale from the inhaler tube, count 1 to 5 slowly as you inhale. The EO molecules get drawn into our bloodstream through our nasal cavity and gets delivered throughout our entire body.

Simple to use, easy to cary, portable and compact. You never have to be without your favorite blends, ever.

Inhaler Blending Basics

Inhalers are super easy and simple to make.

All you need is an inhaler set which consist of the following:

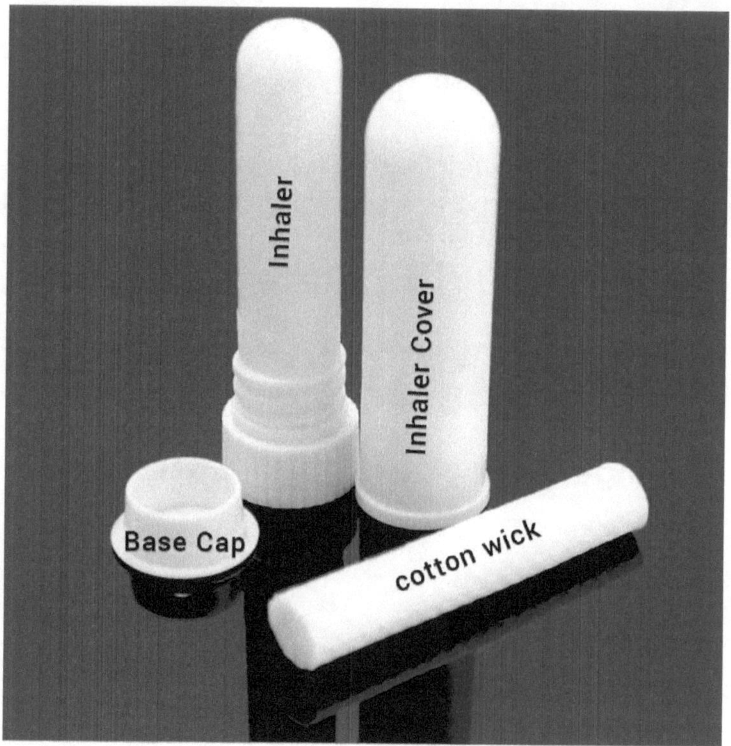

Inhaler, Inhaler Cover, Base Cap and Cotton Wick.

You will need your Essential Oils.

I like to use a pipette for precision and a small petri dish so I can see the oil.

Blending is super easy, just combine the drops and swirl it around in the petri dish and when you are satisfied you can go ahead and drop the cotton wick to absorb all the oil in the dish.

Once the wick is ready you can drop it in the inhaler and cap the bottom with the Base Cap. I usually like to secure the cover with the inhaler so I don't have to do it later.

I usually us 15-20 drops of EO total in a recipe and it can last up to 3 months. Some recipes will need more but on average it is in this range.

Inhaler Recipes

3 drops of Peppermint
3 drops of Rosemary
3 drops of Lime
3 drops of Lemon
3 drops of Grapefruit

----

10 drops of Clary Sage
3 drops of Frankincense
3 drops of Peppermint

----

4 drops of White Fir
3 drops of Grapefruit
3 drops of Orange
2 drops of Lemon
2 drops of Tangerine
1 drop of Bergamot

----

5 drops of Bergamot
4 drops of Orange
3 drops of White Fir
3 drops of Geranium

----

4 drops of Black Pepper
4 drops of Lime
4 drops of Orange
3 drops of Frankincense

----

5 drops of Bergamot
4 drops of Tangerine

3 drops of Basil
3 drops of Clary Sage

----

6 drops of Geranium
6 drops of Rose
3 drops of Ylang Ylang

----

5 drops of Frankincense
4 drops of Ylang Ylang
3 drops of Sandalwood
3 drops of Patchouli

----

6 drops of Tangerine
4 drops of Juniper
3 drops of Bergamot
2 drops of Clary Sage

----

4 drops of Cinnamon
4 drops of Balsam Fir
2 drops of Peppermint
5 drops of Orange

----

4 drops of Dill
3 drops of Fennel
4 drops of Lavender
4 drops of Lemongrass

----

4 drops of Geranium
4 drops of Lemon
2 drops of Ylang Ylang

----

4 drops of Bergamot
4 drops of Juniper Berry
3 drops of Frankincense
3 drops of Peppermint
3 drops of Rosemary
3 drops of Lime
3 drops of Lemon
3 drops of Grapefruit

----

10 drops of Clary Sage
3 drops of Frankincense
3 drops of Peppermint

----

4 drops of White Fir
3 drops of Grapefruit
3 drops of Orange
2 drops of Lemon
2 drops of Tangerine
1 drop of Bergamot

----

5 drops of Bergamot
4 drops of Orange
3 drops of White Fir
3 drops of Geranium

----

4 drops of Black Pepper
4 drops of Lime
4 drops of Orange
3 drops of Frankincense

----

5 drops of Bergamot
4 drops of Tangerine
3 drops of Basil
3 drops of Clary Sage

----

6 drops of Geranium
6 drops of Rose
3 drops of Ylang Ylang

----

5 drops of Frankincense
4 drops of Ylang Ylang
3 drops of Sandalwood
3 drops of Patchouli

----

6 drops of Tangerine
4 drops of Juniper
3 drops of Bergamot
2 drops of Clary Sage

----

4 drops of Cinnamon
4 drops of Balsam Fir
2 drops of Peppermint
5 drops of Orange

----

4 drops of Dill
3 drops of Fennel
4 drops of Lavender
4 drops of Lemongrass

----

4 drops of Geranium
4 drops of Lemon
2 drops of Ylang Ylang

----

4 drops of Bergamot
4 drops of Juniper Berry
3 drops of Frankincense

----

5 drops of Wild Orange
5 drops of Bergamot
5 drops of Sandalwood
5 drops of Ylang Ylang

----

10 drops of Vetiver
6 drops of Sandalwood or Cedarwood
5 drops of Ylang Ylang

----

4 drops of Ylang Ylang
7 drops of Orange
4 drops of Lavender

----

6 drops of Lemon
2 drops of Basil
2 drops of Rosemary
2 drops of Frankincense

----

6 drops of Lavender
3 drops of Lemon
3 drops of Ylang Ylang

----

10 drops of Roman Chamomile
5 drops of Lavender
3 drops of Vetiver

----

10 drops of Palmarosa
5 drops of Geranium
5 drops of Lavender

----

4 drops Lavender
4 drops Orange
4 drops Frankincense
3 drops Cedarwood

----

6 drops Lavender
5 drops Lime
4 drops Spearmint

----

8 drops of Lavender
4 drops of Roman Chamomile

----

5 drops of Frankincense
4 drops of Ylang Ylang
3 drops of Sandalwood
3 drops of Patchouli

----

6 drops of Tangerine
4 drops of Juniper
3 drops of Bergamot
2 drops of Clary Sage

Book Ordering

To order your copy / copies of
Essential Oils for Depression

please visit: **EOrecipes.net**

You can also check out other titles available.

Bulk Pricing and Affiliate Programs Available